YOU CAN REVERSE DEMENTIA

HOW TO RESTORE MEMORY, BOOST MENTAL CLARITY, AND REVERSE COGNITIVE DECLINE AND ALZHEIMER'S

Paul Wayne Bowman

DISCLAIMER

The information expressed in this book is intended to be used for educational purposes only. The author and publisher are not rendering medical advice of any kind, nor is this information to replace medical advice, nor to diagnose, prescribe or treat any disease, condition, illness or injury.

It is imperative that before beginning any nutrition or exercise program you receive full medical clearance from a licensed healthcare professional. The author and publisher claim no responsibility to any person or entity for any liability, loss, or damage caused or alleged to be caused directly or indirectly as a result of the use, application, or interpretation of the material in this book.

Heads up! This book contains **affiliate links.** If you choose to make a purchase through one of them, I may earn a small commission at no extra cost to you. I only recommend products I genuinely believe will be helpful. Being an affiliate will never sway what I recommend or where I recommend getting it.

Introduction

This book is for **you**.

I have written this as if I was speaking to you. You may be experiencing cognitive decline, or you may be a caregiver, partner, child, or friend. I see you, and I understand that you are likely facing the hardest challenge of your life.

To the caregivers, partners, children, and friends reading this: Your role is vital, and the strategies within these pages are designed to be a roadmap for the whole team.

Whether you picked up this book in hope, fear, or weary determination, please know this: you are not alone, and you are right to be looking for answers. The diagnosis of 'dementia' or 'cognitive decline' can feel like a final sentence, but I am here to tell you that it is not the end of the story.

This journey requires courage, patience, and a willingness to try a new path. For the person reading this who wants to reclaim their memory and independence, I will be your guide. For the loved one who is providing support, I will give you the tools and knowledge to be the most effective partner possible. Together, we are going to explore the research and strategies that demonstrate that cognitive function is far more resilient than we have been led to believe.

FYI. This is the same exact protocol I would recommend for preventing dementia.

Prologue

Why I Had to Write This Book

My family's story is why this book exists.

My grandmother, my dad's mother, passed away from dementia. As I write this, my uncle, my dad's brother, is in a nursing home suffering from severe cognitive decline. My dad is rightfully concerned, determined to do everything in his power to prevent this disease from claiming him. Helping him not just survive, but **thrive**, is mission of mine.

I also carry my own high risk.

I was born with no fear, plus cravings for speed, heights, and impact, which resulted in over **100 concussions** across the first 22 years of my life—from falling out of trees to hockey, martial arts, and reckless snow skiing. This family history, combined with my own history of traumatic brain injury, puts me squarely in the high-risk category for cognitive decline.

When I discovered the field of neuro-rehabilitation, it wasn't just a career; it was an obsession. I knew it was the missing piece of our fitness and medical world, and I knew I needed it just as much as the people I worked with.

But here is the most important truth: **99% of people who receive a diagnosis of dementia or Alzheimer's will hear some version of, "There is not much we can do."**

That sentence is **no longer true.** The word must get out.

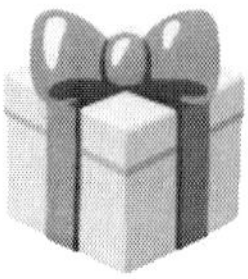

Your 7-Day QuickStart Guide to Reversal of Cognitive Decline

Get Instant Access Now

https://youcanreversedementia.com/quickstart

Table of Contents

CHAPTER 1

THE NEW REALITY

WHY REVERSAL IS POSSIBLE

The vast majority will still say something like, "Dementia is a progressive, degenerative disease that cannot be reversed."

That is clearly no longer true. Dementia, Alzheimer's and cognitive decline have been being reversed for several years.

"All truth passes through three stages. First, it is ridiculed. Second, it is violently opposed. Third, it is accepted as being self-evident" Arthur Schopenhauer

Medicine is always changing. The medical community's main focus since the discovery of dementia has been and still is to cure it with a drug or combination of drugs. They have been able to slow the decline, but have not been able to stop or reverse it.

Thankfully there were a few people out there that started thinking, "What are all the things in life that make a brain healthy? Let's try that."

And…

The most significant and conclusive studies point to multi-faceted lifestyle interventions as the most effective and evidence-based approach to improving and maintaining cognitive function for the prevention or reversal of dementia or Alzheimer's.

At first these studies were ridiculed. But the studies got better. Better done. Better documented. Better able to counter the ridicule.

We are now at a place where most of the world still believes that dementia is irreversible. But there are a handful of relatively small circles of people that know this is no longer true. It is time to spread the word and make it common knowledge. Shout it from the rooftops. "You can prevent and reverse dementia!"

New dementia cases are growing exponentially. It is time to turn that around so another human being and their family do not have to go through the agony of someone losing their mind.

Let me be really clear and transparent in what I'm saying. When people with mild cognitive decline and a diagnosis of dementia or Alzheimer's adopt a lifestyle that supports brain health, roughly 70% will see significant improvement in cognition and other dementia/Alzheimer's symptoms.

There are cases where people have moderate decline as well as severe decline that have seen significant improvement. That said, the further that decline gets, the less likely that someone's going to see a change or a significant improvement.

And I would just say that comes down to resources—resources for that person, and resources for their caregivers. At some point, you're just unable to turn things around.

But the earlier you catch it, the more you work on your lifestyle, the better your odds are of making significant improvements. And you do see people go from mild cognitive impairment to what's considered normal. You see people go from moderate to mild, and in rare cases, you see even more.

What follows are the pieces that make up a healthy brain lifestyle for preventing or reversing dementia.

CHAPTER 2

HEALTHCARE PROFESSIONAL

If you have not already done so, check in with your healthcare professional.

Make sure to rule out or address any of the following potential causes of cognitive decline.

- Infection
- Prescription or over the counter drugs (see next chapter)
- Depression
- Vitamin B12 Deficiency
- Hypothyroidism
- Sleep Apnea
- Alcoholism

CHAPTER 3

PHARMACEUTICALS TO AVOID

Drugs Linked to Dementia Risk

A number of medications have been linked to an increased risk of cognitive decline and dementia, particularly with long-term use and in older adults who may metabolize drugs differently. It's crucial to understand that while these drugs may be associated with an increased risk, it doesn't mean they will cause dementia in every individual, and sometimes the benefits of the medication outweigh the potential risks. Always consult with a healthcare professional before making any changes to your medication regimen.

Here are some of the main classes of drugs that have been associated with dementia or cognitive impairment:

- Anticholinergic Drugs: These drugs block the action of acetylcholine, a neurotransmitter important for memory, attention, and learning. Many common medications have anticholinergic properties.
    - Examples:
        - Antihistamines: Diphenhydramine (Benadryl), doxylamine (Unisom)
        - Tricyclic Antidepressants: Amitriptyline (Elavil), doxepin, nortriptyline (Pamelor)

    - Bladder Control Medications: Oxybutynin (Ditropan), tolterodine (Detrol), fesoterodine (Toviaz)
    - Antipsychotics: Quetiapine (Seroquel), risperidone (Risperdal)
    - Antiparkinson Drugs: Benztropine, trihexyphenidyl
    - Muscle Relaxants: Cyclobenzaprine
    - Gastrointestinal Antispasmodics
- Benzodiazepines: These tranquilizers are prescribed for anxiety, insomnia, panic disorders, and seizures. They can cause sedation and impair memory.
    - Examples: Alprazolam (Xanax), chlordiazepoxide (Librium), clonazepam (Klonopin), diazepam (Valium), lorazepam (Ativan), temazepam (Restoril)
- "Z-drugs" (Non-Benzodiazepine Hypnotics): These sleep aids have similar effects to benzodiazepines.
    - Examples: Zolpidem (Ambien), eszopiclone (Lunesta), zaleplon (Sonata)
- Proton Pump Inhibitors (PPIs): Used to treat acid reflux and ulcers. Some studies suggest a link to dementia, possibly due to affecting vitamin B12 absorption or promoting amyloid plaque buildup.

    - Examples: Omeprazole (Prilosec), lansoprazole (Prevacid), esomeprazole (Nexium)

- Pain Relievers:
    - Opioids: Can cause short-term memory loss and have a high potential for addiction.
    - NSAIDs (Non-Steroidal Anti-inflammatory Drugs): While some studies have explored a potential protective effect of NSAIDs against Alzheimer's, others suggest a higher risk for older adults with long-term use, possibly due to increased risk of internal bleeding. (e.g., ibuprofen, naproxen).
    - Acetaminophen (Paracetamol): Some studies have also included acetaminophen in associations with increased dementia risk, though more research is needed to fully understand the mechanisms.
- Anticonvulsants: Used to treat seizures. They can depress central nervous system activity, potentially affecting memory.
- Certain Antidepressants: While some antidepressants (especially SSRIs) may be used to manage behavioral symptoms of dementia, some types, particularly tricyclic antidepressants (which have anticholinergic properties), have been linked to cognitive issues.

- Statins: Cholesterol-lowering medications. Some research suggests they may impair memory by lowering cholesterol levels in the brain, though other research suggests potential benefits for brain health. The evidence on statins and dementia risk is mixed and continues to be studied.
- Antipsychotics: Used to treat psychosis and manage behavioral difficulties, particularly in the elderly. Atypical antipsychotics, while sometimes used for dementia-related agitation, carry a warning about an increased risk of death in older patients with dementia-related psychosis.

Important Considerations:

- Dosage and Duration: The risk often increases with higher doses and longer durations of use.
- Polypharmacy: Taking multiple medications simultaneously, especially those with similar side effects, can increase the risk of cognitive impairment.
- Individual Differences: How a medication affects an individual can vary based on age, overall health, genetics, and how their body metabolizes drugs.
- Reversibility: In some cases, medication-induced cognitive decline can be reversible if the offending drug is discontinued or the dosage is reduced under medical supervision. This is often referred to as "pseudodementia" when the cognitive issues resemble dementia.

It is crucial for individuals, especially older adults, to regularly review all their medications (prescription and over-the-counter) with their healthcare provider to identify any potential risks and discuss safer alternatives if necessary. It is important to realize that this is usually NOT done automatically.

CHAPTER 4

ASSESS

Sage

MoCA

AARP Staying Sharp

Here are three assessments to take to get a good baseline to compare to in the future.

Sage

One of the most widely recognized and scientifically validated self-assessments is the Self-Administered Gerocognitive Examination (SAGE). It is a paper-and-pencil test developed by researchers at The Ohio State University Wexner Medical Center.

Here's why the SAGE test is often recommended:

- Purpose: It is designed to detect early signs of mild cognitive impairment (MCI) and early dementia.
- Content: The test assesses multiple cognitive domains, including orientation, language, reasoning, memory, visuospatial function, and executive function.

- Accessibility: It can be taken at home and is available in four interchangeable forms to reduce "practice effects" if taken multiple times.
- Next Steps: After completing the test, you take your results to a doctor for scoring and interpretation. The score helps the doctor determine if further evaluation is necessary.

https://wexnermedical.osu.edu/brain-spine-neuro/memory-disorders/sage

You can download a mobile app version of the SAGE test at https://Braintest.com

If you choose this option, you will need to sign up for their free 30-day trial. You can then immediately take the 15-minute test. And you will get your results the next day. Then remember to cancel your trial membership unless you wish to continue with them.

MoCA

Have a friend or loved one, administer the Montreal Cognitive Assessment (MoCA). It takes about 10 minutes.

https://www.mdcalc.com/calc/10044/montreal-cognitive-assessment-moca

There are three versions, so you can repeat it without concern that any improvement comes from having seen the same test before. A normal MoCA score is 26 to 30; 19 to 25 is associated with MCI;

19–22, if accompanied by difficulties with activities of daily living, usually means that MCI has converted to dementia, whether from Alzheimer's disease or another cause; and scores lower than 19 indicate dementia.

AARP Staying Sharp

This assessment measures speed and accuracy in five key areas: processing speed, attention, working memory, cognitive flexibility, and recognition memory. It's free for AARP members and registered users of their website. You can sign up for a free AARP membership. The results are compared to others of the same age, gender, and education level. https://stayingsharp.aarp.org/

The AARP Staying Sharp Cognitive Assessment and the associated Lifestyle Check-Ins are designed to be completed together and take approximately 40 minutes. It's recommended that you find a quiet place with no distractions to complete them in a single sitting.

There are also "Additional Tests" that can be taken after the main assessment, which may take up to 20 minutes to complete. These tests explore other cognitive elements like nonverbal reasoning and spatial processing.

If you are interrupted or need to step away, you can typically pick up where you left off for up to an hour before you may need to start over.

AARP members and users with an aarp.org account can take the Cognitive Assessment, Lifestyle Check-Ins and Additional Tests for FREE. And you can take the Assessment every 30 days at no cost.

I encourage you to take all three and then retake these about every three months after adopting a healthy brain lifestyle.

CHAPTER 5

FOOD

A healthy brain needs fuel and stimulation.

Fuel = Food + Breath

Dementia has been reversed with the Ketogenic Diet, the Mediterranean Diet, as well as a clean balanced diet that provides all your nutrition.

My preference is the clean balanced diet that provides all your nutrition.

Clean means:

- No Fast Food
- No Junk Food
- Foods that are not processed or are minimally processed
- No artificial sweeteners
- No artificial flavors
- No processing agents

Here are your targets for a balanced diet that provides all your nutrition.

Macro Targets

Protein: .7-1.2g/lb. of bodyweight per day

Fat: 10-20% of your dietary calories

Carbohydrates: The remainder of your calories should come from carbohydrates. To better understand some common misconceptions about carbs and sugar, make sure to read the Diabetes chapter.

Vitamin and Mineral Targets: Unless you are taking more for a specific reason, your target is the DV (Daily Value)

A great tool for tracking all this is Cronometer.

Get the free version of https://cronometer.com/ or another food app that does the same thing.
Journal all your food, drink, and supplements for a few weeks or until you are confident that you are getting a great balance of all your macros, vitamins and minerals.
Cronometer has an online version and a mobile app version that will sync in real time. I prefer the online version for most things. The mobile app is great for scanning bar codes.

Grains
I recommend eliminating grains. Grains are a big contributor to inflammation which is a big contributor to dementia.

Eggs

A recent study of 1,024 people showed that eating at least one egg per week reduced the risk of Alzheimer's by 47%.

Remember that too much of a good thing is not always a good thing. I do not recommend more than 7 eggs per week.

CHAPTER 6

FAT SOLUBLE VITAMINS A,D,E,K

The comprehensive nutritional demands of a healing brain go far beyond simply avoiding fast food; they require precision. To truly rebuild cognitive function, we must ensure every critical building block is present in the right amounts. Among the most essential components are the fat-soluble vitamins A, D, E, and K. Because they are absorbed with fat and stored in the body's tissues, they play non-negotiable roles in hormone production, immune regulation, blood clotting, and, most importantly, the structural integrity of your neurons. Here are my recommendations for achieving and maintaining optimal levels of these critical four.

Vitamin A would be best from 4 ounces of grass-fed beef liver per week. Liver is the most nutrient dense food there is. I put it in a crock pot of stew, so I do not taste it at all. Publix supermarkets have a grass-fed liver in the freezer section. Whole Foods has a great ground beef with organ meat. If not that, then grab Simply A. Vitamin A (as Retinol) supplementation should be 4-8 times that of Vitamin D3 supplementation.

https://healthnatura.com/simply-a-2-500-i-u-1oz/?ref=neurocoachnaplesfl

Vitamin D3: Get enough healthy sunshine and supplementation to get your Vitamin D, 25-OH, D3 blood test between 50-60 ng/ml.

https://amzn.to/4q7YzQm

Vitamin E: Vitamin E is a powerful antioxidant that protects cells from damage caused by free radicals, which can contribute to chronic diseases such as cancer, heart disease, and Alzheimer's disease.

https://www.amazon.com/dp/B000SAXU0Y

Vitamin K2: K2 is the biggest determiner of where digested minerals go. 5 mg 3 times per day. Or up to 15 mg 3 times per day for high blood pressure or osteoporosis. If you are on any blood thinners, check with your healthcare professional before taking vitamin K2.

https://healthnatura.com/true-k2-mk4-1-mg-per-drop-1-ounce/?ref=neurocoachnaplesfl

CHAPTER 7

HORMONES

Hormones are the body's chemical messengers, regulating everything from your metabolism and sleep cycle to your mood and stress response. When seeking to reverse dementia, you must pay close attention to your endocrine system, as imbalances in key hormones can accelerate cognitive decline, while restoring balance can provide a powerful, therapeutic boost to your brain.

The following are all produced by the body, but that production slows down as you age.

Pregnenolone protects brain cells from injury caused by fatigue.

DHEA blocks the destructive effects of excess cortisone caused by chronic stress and actively restores the normal growth and repair processes.

Experiments have shown that progesterone relieves anxiety, improves memory, protects brain cells, and even prevents epileptic seizures.

Pregnenolone: 50mg/day

https://healthnatura.com/pregnenolone-20-grams/?ref=neurocoachnaplesfl

DHEA: 4 drops per day

https://amzn.to/48sgbQG

Progesterone: 14 drops

https://healthnatura.com/simply-progesterone-1-08-oz/?ref=neurocoachnaplesfl

CHAPTER 8

CREATINE

Creatine, a compound naturally produced by the body, in food, and as a supplement, is well-known for its role in athletic performance. However, a growing body of research highlights its significant benefits for brain health, primarily by improving the brain's energy supply.

Here's a summary of the benefits of creatine for brain health:

- Improved Cognitive Function: Creatine supplementation has been shown to enhance cognitive functions, particularly in areas of short-term memory, intelligence, and reasoning. These effects are often most pronounced in individuals under metabolic stress, such as older adults, those with sleep deprivation, or individuals with certain neurological conditions.
- Enhanced Brain Energy: The brain is a highly energy-demanding organ, consuming about 20% of the body's energy. Creatine plays a crucial role in brain bioenergetics by helping to maintain stable levels of ATP (adenosine triphosphate), the primary energy molecule used by cells. By increasing brain creatine stores, supplementation can help ensure a steady energy supply for complex mental tasks, potentially reducing mental fatigue.

- Neuroprotection: Creatine may help protect nerve cells from injury or damage. It has shown promise in improving recovery and health outcomes associated with conditions like traumatic brain injury and muscular dystrophy. Creatine may also play a role in reducing inflammation and oxidative stress, which are major factors in brain aging and neurodegenerative diseases.

- Potential for Neurological Conditions: While more research is needed, preliminary studies suggest creatine may be beneficial for individuals with specific neurological conditions. For example, a pilot study on Alzheimer's patients found moderate improvements in working memory and executive function. Creatine has also shown potential for reducing symptoms of depression and anxiety.

10 g per day is the typical dose for brain health. Spread through the day is best. Too much at once can cause loose or watery stool. Many will take 15-20 g throughout the day if they had a poor night's sleep.

https://amzn.to/4q6WlR7

CHAPTER 9

BREATH

The goal here is to have good breathing habits, so that you get the best balance of oxygen and CO2.

Most of us in modern society are chronically stressed to varying degrees and this is reflected in how we breathe. The more stressed and the more sedentary we become, the more likely we are chest breathers, mouth breathers, and our CO2 tolerance is getting lower and lower.

CO2 is not just a waste gas as we were taught in our elementary education. CO2 being high enough is the trigger to get oxygen to our tissues.

When you are relaxed, how many breaths per minute do you take? It should be less than 14.

What is your BOLT score? Exhale and hold your breath until you have an urge to breathe. NOT as long as you can, but until you have an urge to breath which will be a spasm of the diaphragm or throat. Healthy is considered 40 seconds or greater. This test is a good indication of your CO2 tolerance.

To make changes in your autonomic breathing takes at least 20 minutes per day of practice. This could be all at once or broken up.

If you are a mouth breather, practice nose breathing.

If you are a chest breather, practice using your entire torso, expanding and contracting your entire rib cage, belly, low back, and diaphragm.

If you are breathing too quickly, practice slowing it down.

If you have a low BOLT score, practice your exhale holds and be patient.

CHAPTER 10

MOVEMENT

For a healthy brain, move well and move often.

To stay healthy, the brain needs fuel and stimulation. Quality movement is the best stimulation you can give your brain.

Quality movement means movement that you enjoy and that is making you better in ways that matter to you.

A minimum here would be 30-35 minutes of moderate-to-intense aerobic activity four times a week, plus strength and flexibility exercises twice a week. And moderate-to-intense is relative to you. Do your best and your best gets better.

Do your best not to be sedentary for more than an hour or two. Get some quality movement for at least 2 minutes every 90 minutes.

CHAPTER 11

STIMULATION

A healthy brain needs fuel and stimulation.

In addition to movement, stimulation would involve all of your senses.

Sight

In modern society most people do not move their eyes the way we should.

So, I encourage you to move your eyes as often as you can safely. And short of strain or fatigue. Look up, down, left, right, and into the corners. Get outside. Look far and near. Let your eyes follow things: children, birds, dogs, cars…Practice using your peripheral vision. Practice holding your gaze on something while you move your head and body.

Proper red-light therapy has been shown to help most common eye diseases. https://www.instagram.com/reel/DKokOkdg5Ix/

It is possible to stop and reverse most vision loss with proper nutrition, red light, exercises, etc.

Hearing

Have you had your hearing checked recently or at all? I suggest that you do. And get the hearing aids if needed. And wear the hearing aids. And get the settings professionally personalized. And get trained in how to use them. It all matters (to your brain).

Whenever you think of it, practice using your hearing. What do you hear? Where is the sound coming from?

Smell

Humans have about 400 receptors for smell. Using them is vital to your brain health.

With just their sense of smell, natives can identify many species of animals and plants. And not just identify but can tell you specifics about the plant or animal they smell.

As domesticated humans we have lost most of those skills. And as we age we tend to use our senses less and less. Use it or lose it.

Stop and smell the flowers. Stop and smell everything.

Can you smell it and can you identify it is a good game to play with a friend or family member.

Sometimes use your left nostril. Sometimes use your right nostril. Sometimes use both.

Taste

When eating, pause and really taste your food. Smell your food.

Regularly get a variety of healthy flavors in your food.

Touch

Ideally you would experience the whole spectrum of touch every day.

- Warm
- Cool
- Light Touch
- Heavy Touch
- Vibration
- Sharp (safely)(example: getting your back scratched)
- Chemical (safely)(examples: menthol, peppermint)

CHAPTER 12

COGNITIVE EXERCISE

Sharpening the Mind

Both physical exercise and cognitive exercise strengthen your brain. Cognitive exercise promotes the growth of new connections and enhances the brain's ability to rewire itself—a process known as neuroplasticity. For those seeking to reverse dementia, engaging the brain in challenging, novel activities is not a mere pastime; it's a form of targeted therapy.

The Science of a Plastic Brain

Decades of research have overturned the old belief that the adult brain is a fixed entity. The brain is remarkably adaptable, and you can harness this adaptability to improve cognitive function.

1. Neuroplasticity: The Brain's Ability to Rewire

Neuroplasticity is the core mechanism behind cognitive exercise. It allows the brain to reorganize itself by forming new neural connections throughout life. When you learn a new skill or challenge your mind, you are literally:

- Growing New Neurons (Neurogenesis): Primarily in the hippocampus, the brain's memory center.

- Strengthening Synapses: Making existing connections faster and more efficient. This is the biological basis of learning and memory consolidation.
- Creating "Cognitive Reserve": Building a robust network of alternate neural pathways. The greater your cognitive reserve, the more resilient your brain is to damage caused by diseases like Alzheimer's, effectively allowing you to continue functioning normally even if some brain regions are compromised.

2. The Use-It-or-Lose-It Principle

The brain follows a simple but strict rule: connections that are used get stronger, and those that aren't get weaker.

- Novelty is Key: Repetitive, routine tasks (like the same old daily crossword puzzle) require less brain power over time. For cognitive exercise to be effective, it must involve novelty and be mentally demanding.
- Challenging Multiple Domains: The most effective cognitive exercises challenge different areas of the brain simultaneously: memory, executive function (planning, decision-making), and speed of processing.

The Three Pillars of Effective Cognitive Exercise

To maximize neuroplasticity and build cognitive reserve, your routine should incorporate activities from these three key categories: Learning, Socializing, and Creative Expression.

Pillar 1: Challenging New Learning (Novelty)

This is the most powerful category because it forces the brain to build entirely new circuits. The activity should be complex and push you outside your comfort zone.

- Learn a Foreign Language: This is often cited as the *ultimate* brain exercise. It demands proficiency in listening, speaking, reading, writing, grammar, vocabulary, and memory, engaging widespread neural networks.
- Master a New Musical Instrument: Playing an instrument engages the auditory cortex, motor cortex, and visual-spatial processing areas all at once, leading to significant and widespread structural changes in the brain.
- Take a College-Level Course: Enroll in a class on physics, history, philosophy, or coding. The act of synthesizing complex new information is a high-level cognitive workout.
- Learn a Complex, Multi-Step Craft: Activities like knitting, complex cooking, wood carving, or intricate carpentry require executive function, planning, and fine motor skills.

Pillar 2: Strategic Play and Engagement (Mental Agility)

These activities improve speed, attention, and problem-solving skills, which are often the first to decline.

- Strategic Games: Play games that require deep strategy and forward planning, such as Chess, Go, or Bridge. These games train your executive function and working memory.
- Novel Puzzles: Go beyond simple crosswords. Try Sudoku, complex jigsaws, logic puzzles, or non-routine math problems to challenge your speed and reasoning.
- "Brain Training" Apps (Use with Caution): While some targeted apps can help with specific skills like attention, they should not replace real-world challenging activities. Use them as a supplement, focusing on modules that feel genuinely difficult.
- Become a Tech Wizard: Learn to use a new software program, edit a video, or build a website. These tasks require novel problem-solving and focus.

Pillar 3: Socializing and Creative Expression (Connection)

Engaging with others and expressing yourself creatively provides a crucial mix of emotional, cognitive, and social stimulation.

- Social Connection: Join a book club, a debate group, or a dance class. Robust social interaction is a complex cognitive activity involving interpreting language, body language, emotional cues, and keeping track of conversation threads.
- Creative Writing/Journaling: Writing fiction, poetry, or detailed personal narratives engages language centers and

requires the brain to organize abstract thought into concrete structure.

- Art and Sculpture: Engaging in visual arts—painting, drawing, sculpting—activates areas related to visual processing, motor control, and creative problem-solving.
- Improvisation and Drama: Participating in acting or improv classes is an exceptional workout for executive function, as you must rapidly recall information, make split-second decisions, and respond flexibly to unpredictable situations.

Integration: Your Personalized Cognitive Prescription

Cognitive exercise should be integrated into your life, not viewed as a separate chore. Think of it as enriching your environment to make your brain work harder and smarter every day.

Principle	Actionable Tip
Combine Skills	If you are learning a language, talk with native speakers (social + learning). If you are learning an instrument, play in a band (motor + social).
Increase Difficulty	Once an activity becomes easy, increase the challenge. Learn a new defense strategy in chess, or move from basic vocabulary to complex literature in your new language.
Mindfulness and Focus	Be present during the activity. If your mind wanders, gently bring it back. The cognitive benefit comes from the focused struggle.
Consistency Over Intensity	Aim for small, consistent efforts every day. Ten minutes of focused language practice is better than a three-hour marathon once a month.

By prioritizing mentally stimulating, novel, and challenging activities, you actively push your brain to grow, creating a powerful defense against cognitive decline and charting a strong course toward reversing its effects.

At least 3 times per week for 30 minutes challenge your cognition.

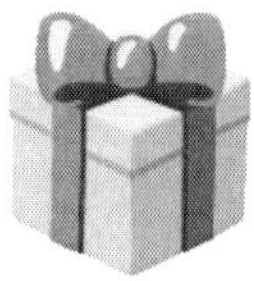

Your 7-Day QuickStart Guide to Reversal of Cognitive Decline

Get Instant Access Now

https://youcanreversedementia.com/quickstart

CHAPTER 13

CHOLESTEROL

A meta-analysis of all the well-done studies on this subject now shows that the longest living healthiest people have an average total cholesterol of 225-270.

Cholesterol is an essential building block for everything in our bodies. A total cholesterol of less than 150, especially when artificially lowered by something like statins, contributes to brain degeneration as well as other problems.

LDL is only bad when it is oxidized. Big culprits for this are trans fats, polyunsaturated fats (PUFA) (Vegetable oil, fish oil, nuts, seeds), and smoking.

The Brain Health world is divided on whether PUFA is good or bad. I am on team minimize PUFA as much as possible. My argument in this debate revolves around "healthier" vs "healthy". The jump is often made from something being a healthier option to then being deemed healthy. In this case are Omega 3's less inflammatory than Omega 6's? Yes, but I would say that does not justify deeming them healthy. Polyunsaturated fats (PUFAs) are chemically unstable and more prone to oxidation than other types of fats. High levels of oxidation cause cell damage, which leads to dysfunction, premature aging, and a variety of diseases including dementia.

If LDL or any cholesterol is high in the blood, that means it is not getting processed and not getting to where it needs to be in the body. The biggest culprits for this are low Vitamin A, Low Vitamin D or low thyroid.

CHAPTER 14

DEPRESSION

Depression is more than just feeling sad; it's a serious medical condition that significantly interacts with and accelerates cognitive decline. For those seeking to reverse dementia, treating depression is not a secondary goal—it is a primary, therapeutic intervention. Unmanaged depression can mimic the symptoms of dementia, worsen the progression of underlying disease, and sabotage your commitment to the demanding lifestyle changes required for reversal.

The Vicious Cycle: Depression and Dementia

The relationship between depression and dementia is complex, with each condition fueling the other in a detrimental cycle.

1. Depression as a Risk Factor

Research overwhelmingly shows that depression, particularly when experienced earlier in life or in midlife, dramatically increases the risk of developing dementia later on.

- Neuro-Inflammation: Depression is closely linked to chronic, systemic inflammation—the same destructive process that damages neurons and accelerates the formation of amyloid plaques and tau tangles.

- Stress Hormone Overload: Depression activates the HPA axis, leading to persistently high levels of cortisol. This hormone is toxic to the hippocampus, the brain's memory center, worsening atrophy and impairing memory formation.
- Structural Changes: Long-term depression is associated with a reduction in the volume of the hippocampus and other crucial brain structures.

2. Depression as a Symptom

Conversely, depression is often an early symptom of the underlying brain changes that cause dementia. The disease process itself—the accumulation of plaques and tangles—can begin years before noticeable memory loss, manifesting first as changes in mood, apathy, or anxiety.

3. Depression Mimicking Dementia (Pseudodementia)

In some cases, severe depression in older adults can present with such profound cognitive impairment (memory loss, slow thinking, apathy) that it is mistakenly diagnosed as dementia. This condition is sometimes referred to as pseudodementia. Successfully treating the depression in these individuals often leads to a complete reversal of the cognitive symptoms. This underscores why treating the mood disorder is essential for accurate diagnosis and effective reversal.

The Cognitive Costs of Depression

Depression directly impairs the cognitive functions you are trying to restore:

- Apathy and Motivation: Depression drains motivation, making it nearly impossible to consistently adhere to the rigorous diet, exercise, cognitive stimulation, and stress management protocols necessary for reversal.
- Executive Dysfunction: It impairs the prefrontal cortex, leading to poor executive function—difficulty with planning, decision-making, focus, and organizing tasks.
- Sleep Disruption: Depression and poor sleep are inextricably linked. Sleep is when the brain clears out neurotoxic proteins via the glymphatic system. Depressive sleep disturbances (insomnia or excessive sleeping) severely hinder this crucial nightly "brain wash."

Your Action Plan for Mood and Cognitive Recovery

Treating depression requires a holistic approach that integrates lifestyle and medical interventions.

1. Optimize Foundational Reversal Protocols

The core elements of your reversal plan are powerful mood stabilizers.

- Physical Exercise: Regular aerobic and resistance exercise is one of the most effective and accessible anti-depressants. It boosts endorphins, increases the growth factor BDNF

(Brain-Derived Neurotrophic Factor), and reduces inflammation.

- Dietary Intervention: There is a growing body of evidence suggesting that nutrition plays a significant role in mental health, including depression. Studies have shown that nutrient deficiencies may be associated with an increased risk of developing depression, while addressing those deficiences may have protective effects.
- Social Connection: Combat the isolation that feeds depression. As discussed in the previous chapter, meaningful social engagement provides purpose, stimulation, and a buffer against stress.

2. Address Underlying Nutritional Deficiencies

Several common nutritional deficiencies are strongly linked to both depression and cognitive decline:

- B Vitamins (B12, Folate): Essential for neurotransmitter production and lowering homocysteine, an inflammatory marker associated with brain atrophy.
- Vitamin D: Low levels are consistently found in depressed patients. Optimization is critical.
- Magnesium: Involved in hundreds of biochemical reactions, including mood and stress regulation.

- Zinc: Low levels can affect immune function and mood stability.

3. Seek Professional and Medical Support

Never attempt to manage clinical depression alone. A dual-diagnosis approach—treating the mood and the cognition simultaneously—is crucial.

- Psychotherapy: Talk therapy, particularly Cognitive Behavioral Therapy (CBT), is highly effective. It helps reframe negative thought patterns and provides coping strategies, restoring a sense of control and self-efficacy.

- Medication: Evaluation: I say this under the umbrella of compassion for anyone struggling with depression, anxiety, or any chronic stress. Medications are not the long-term answer for any of these and may do more harm than good. You may decide that medication could be a good short-term tool while you do the work. If you decide to start or stop any medication, please do so carefully/wisely. But you must do the work. Be patient and love yourself while you do the work.

- Rule Out Other Conditions: Ensure that other medical conditions that can cause depression (e.g., hypothyroidism, anemia, sleep apnea, or hormonal imbalances) have been thoroughly investigated and treated.

By shining a light on and actively treating depression, you not only alleviate emotional suffering but also remove one of the most destructive roadblocks on your path to reversing cognitive decline.

CHAPTER 15

TRAUMATIC BRAIN INJURY (TBI)

If you have ever had head trauma and it was not rehabbed, I encourage you to do the rehab, no matter when that trauma was. Most head traumas are not rehabbed and when they are, rehab is almost always ended too soon.

Head traumas that do not get rehabbed will often creep up on you decades later and can be big contributors to serious brain degeneration.

It is important to realize that most neurologist are excellent at diagnosing, but are not trained in neuro rehab. And most going to a neurologist will never hear about or get referred to neuro rehab. I look forward to a day when neuro prehab and rehab are common.

There are exceptions. If you need it, I hope you are able to work with the exceptions…

- Neurologist that is well trained in neuro rehab
- Functional Neurologist
- Neuro Coach

A Traumatic Brain Injury (TBI), whether a severe blow to the head or a milder concussion, is a significant event that can profoundly impact cognitive health and dramatically increase the risk of dementia. For those working toward cognitive reversal, addressing the lingering effects of a TBI is crucial. This chapter will outline the mechanisms by which TBI fuels neurodegeneration and detail the targeted strategies you can employ to heal the injured brain.

The TBI-Dementia Connection: An Accelerated Risk

A single moderate-to-severe TBI, or multiple concussions, can double or triple the risk of developing dementia, including Alzheimer's disease (AD) and Chronic Traumatic Encephalopathy (CTE).

1. The Cascade of Damage

When the brain sustains an impact, a destructive cascade begins, setting the stage for long-term cognitive problems:

- Acute Inflammation: The initial injury causes immediate, widespread inflammation as the immune system rushes to the site of damage. If this response doesn't shut down, it becomes chronic neuro-inflammation, which is one of the key drivers of dementia.
- Axonal Shearing: TBI causes rapid movement of the brain, leading to the tearing or stretching of nerve fibers (axons). This disrupts communication pathways and can directly damage the cells.
- Vascular Damage: Impact can compromise the blood-brain barrier (BBB), allowing toxins and inflammatory substances from the bloodstream to enter the brain. It also damages

the cerebral vasculature, setting the stage for vascular dementia.

2. Protein Aggregation and Neurodegeneration

TBI acts as a catalyst for the pathological hallmarks of dementia:

- Amyloid and Tau Accumulation: The injury triggers the rapid production and aggregation of beta-amyloid plaques and tau tangles, the characteristic proteins of AD and CTE. Studies show these proteins can begin accumulating immediately after a TBI.
- Mitochondrial Dysfunction: TBI damages the mitochondria (the powerhouses of the cell), leading to a significant energy crisis in the brain. Starved of adequate energy, neurons are unable to perform essential functions, including waste clearance and repair.

Targeted Strategies for TBI-Related Reversal

Healing the TBI-injured brain requires specific interventions. These strategies focus on restoring function to the systems most disrupted by the injury: the visual, vestibular (balance), and cognitive systems.

1. Controlled, Progressive Exercise (Exertion Therapy)

Rest is necessary initially, but prolonged rest is detrimental. Gradual reintroduction of physical activity is a core component of PCS rehab.

- Sub-Symptom Threshold Exercise: Work with a neuro coach to establish your symptom threshold—the level of activity (heart rate) that provokes symptoms like headache or dizziness. Exercise must be performed *below* this threshold.
- Graduated Aerobics: Start with gentle stationary cycling or brisk walking. The goal is to gradually raise the symptom threshold over time, improving cerebral blood flow and boosting the brain-repair factor BDNF (Brain-Derived Neurotrophic Factor) without triggering symptom flare-ups. This carefully managed exercise is vital for both physical and cognitive recovery.

2. Visual/Vestibular and Balance Rehabilitation

TBI often damages the vestibular system, which is responsible for balance and spatial orientation. Correcting this dysfunction is key to reducing dizziness and improving cognitive focus.

Vision is an integral part of your vestibular system. Visual tracking and convergence are often impaired after TBI, leading to difficulties with reading, concentration, and screen time.

- With a behavioral optometrist or neuro coach if needed, rehab: gaze stabilization, smooth pursuits, VORs, VOR-Cs, Convergence, Near/Far, & Saccades.

- Postural Stability: Practice balance exercises, gradually increasing the challenge. This retraining improves the brain's ability to process sensory information.

3. Cognitive Rehabilitation and Pacing

The injured brain struggles with attention and energy management. Cognitive rehab protocols focus on building tolerance and teaching compensatory strategies.

- Pacing and Scheduling: Teach the brain to manage energy by strictly limiting high-demand activities (e.g., computer work, complex meetings) to short, scheduled windows. This prevents the "boom-and-bust" cycle of symptom exacerbation.

- Working Memory Drills: Engage in targeted cognitive exercises (often with a neuro coach or neuropsychologist) to rebuild working memory and processing speed. The key is consistent, controlled exposure to cognitive effort.

- Mindfulness and Stress Management: Integrate techniques like meditation and deep breathing to calm the overactive sympathetic nervous system (fight-or-flight response), which is often perpetually activated after TBI, contributing to headaches, sleep issues, and anxiety.

5. Prioritizing Sleep Hygiene

Since TBI disrupts the brain's sleep-wake cycle and is when the brain clears waste, optimizing sleep is paramount.

- Strict Routine: Maintain a consistent sleep schedule (bedtime and wake-up time).
- Avoid Screens/Stimulants: Eliminate screen time and caffeine/alcohol close to bedtime to allow the brain to naturally transition to rest and repair mode.

By following these structured, progressive rehabilitation protocols, you actively promote neuroplasticity, restore functional balance, and directly address the lingering energy crisis and inflammation caused by TBI, moving you aggressively toward cognitive recovery and reversal.

CHAPTER 16

DIABETIES

Beyond Blood Sugar: Diabetes as "Type 3 Dementia"

For those focused on reversing dementia, Type 2 Diabetes and insulin resistance must be viewed as brain disorders. The strong link between impaired glucose metabolism and cognitive decline has led some researchers to refer to Alzheimer's disease as "Type 3 Diabetes." Controlling and reversing insulin resistance is not just about physical health; it is one of the most powerful and non-negotiable interventions for healing the brain.

The Unbreakable Link: Insulin, Glucose, and the Brain

The brain is the most energy-intensive organ in the body, relying almost exclusively on glucose (sugar) for fuel. The ability of brain cells to use this fuel relies heavily on the hormone insulin.

1. Insulin Resistance: Starving the Neurons

In Type 2 Diabetes and pre-diabetes, the body's cells become resistant to insulin's signal. The pancreas pumps out more and more insulin, but the cells—including those in the brain—simply stop responding.

- Brain Starvation: When brain cells become insulin-resistant, they can no longer efficiently pull glucose from the bloodstream. The brain, which consumes about 20% of the body's energy, enters a state of chronic energy crisis.

- Cognitive Decline: This energy deficit impacts the most demanding cognitive functions first: memory formation, concentration, and executive function. This metabolic dysfunction is a root cause of the fog and memory loss experienced in early cognitive decline.

2. Insulin's Non-Metabolic Role

Insulin doesn't just manage glucose; it also plays a direct, crucial role in neuronal health:

- Synaptic Plasticity: Insulin signaling is essential for neuroplasticity—the brain's ability to create and strengthen new connections, which is the biological basis of learning and memory.

- Amyloid Clearance: Insulin is involved in the process of clearing beta-amyloid (the protein that forms plaques in Alzheimer's disease). When insulin levels are persistently high (hyperinsulinemia), the brain's waste-disposal system gets overwhelmed, accelerating plaque buildup.

3. Sugar and Inflammation

You <u>cannot</u> just say, "Sugar is bad. Sugar causes inflammation." Context matters.

- When sugar comes along with high phycological stress and poor nutrition (chemicals, processing agents, junk oils, missing nutrients, out of balance macro and micronutrients) then it can contribute to things like inflammation, diabetes, and dementia.
- When sugar is part of a clean balanced diet that provides all your nutrition and stress is well managed, sugar is wonderful for your body and brain. Glucose is the preferred fuel source for all cells, especially in the brain. If there is not enough glucose in the diet, the body will break down muscles and organs to get it.

I have helped many rid themselves of their Type 2 diabetes diagnosis.

In doing so, they consumed more sugar than they ever have in the form of things like fruit, juice, honey, maple syrup, and cane sugar. They also had to dial in their nutrition to do this.

By dialing in their nutrition, they were able to lower their blood sugar levels and A1C into the normal range because with the proper nutrition they were able to effectively metabolize glucose, getting it into their cells and fueling their muscles, organs, and brain.

These same ideas can be used for Type 1 Diabetics to reduce their reliance on medications and insulin.

If you are prediabetic, Type 1, or Type 2 I encourage you to read my book, “How to Fix Your Type 2 Diabetes”.

https://payhip.com/b/nOI9p

By actively healing your metabolism, you directly reverse the "Type 3" pathology in your brain, restoring energy and clearing the path for cognitive healing.

CHAPTER 17

HYPERTENSION

The Silent Threat

Hypertension, or high blood pressure, is one of the most common and damaging risk factors for cognitive decline and dementia. It's often called the "silent killer" because it damages blood vessels over years without noticeable symptoms, yet its impact on the brain is profound.

Why Blood Pressure Matters to Your Brain

Your brain is incredibly dependent on a steady, strong flow of oxygen and nutrients delivered via a dense network of tiny blood vessels. When hypertension is present, this vital delivery system is compromised.

1. Vascular Dementia: The Direct Hit

Chronic high blood pressure is the leading cause of vascular dementia. This occurs through several mechanisms:

- Small Vessel Damage: Hypertension causes the small, deep blood vessels in the brain to stiffen, narrow, and become blocked, a condition known as arteriolosclerosis. This starves small clusters of neurons, causing multiple tiny strokes or microinfarcts over time.

- Reduced Blood Flow: Stiffened vessels are less able to regulate blood flow. This constant, high-pressure pounding on the vessel walls damages the delicate lining and impairs the brain's ability to get the oxygen and glucose it needs, particularly in deep brain structures critical for executive function and processing speed.
- White Matter Lesions: High blood pressure damages the white matter (the insulated communication cables connecting different brain regions). This results in lesions that disrupt signal transmission, leading to problems with processing information and difficulty focusing.

2. The Link to Alzheimer's Disease (AD)

Hypertension doesn't just cause vascular dementia; it also accelerates the pathology of Alzheimer's disease.

- Blood-Brain Barrier Compromise: Chronic high blood pressure damages the blood-brain barrier (BBB), allowing inflammatory substances and toxins from the bloodstream to enter the brain and disrupt its sensitive environment.
- Impaired Waste Clearance: The glymphatic system, which clears beta-amyloid plaques and tau tangles (the hallmarks of AD) during sleep, is less efficient when blood vessels are damaged. Hypertension hinders this clearance process, accelerating the buildup of toxic proteins.

Your Action Plan

The evidence is clear: reducing high blood pressure significantly lowers the risk of developing and progressing cognitive decline. Your goal is to not just "treat" hypertension, but to achieve a consistently optimal blood pressure (below 120/80 mmHg).

1. Balance your minerals

- High sodium is not the problem. I wish the context and bigger picture of this were more commonly addressed. Low salt can reduce blood pressure but leads to other problems. Getting enough salt is essential to your health. It only becomes a problem when it is out of balance with other minerals, especially potassium.

- Increase Potassium, Magnesium, and Calcium: Get as much as you can from your diet and supplement if need be. Many common blood pressure medications affect potassium levels, so if you are on any medication consult with your healthcare professional before making any changes.

2. Improve your breathing

- See the “Breath” chapter

3. Exercise

- Isometrics being the best

- Wall sit being the best isometric for lowering blood pressure

4. Stress and Sleep Management

Stress and poor sleep directly spike blood pressure.

- Calm the Sympathetic Nervous System: Use deep breathing exercises, meditation, and mindfulness to activate the parasympathetic nervous system, naturally lowering heart rate and blood pressure.
- Treat Sleep Apnea: Snoring and interrupted breathing during sleep (sleep apnea) cause massive, repeated spikes in blood pressure overnight. Look at raising the head of your bed and mouth taping.

4. Medication

If you decide to start or stop any hypertension drug(s) please do so wisely and safely.

In the long run, hypertension drugs are not the answer to better health or reversing cognitive decline and may do more harm than good.

If you are on one (or more) or decide to go on blood pressure medication, please do your homework and think of it as a short-term solution as you do the work to get healthy.

And neurology can have a huge effect on your blood pressure, so if your high blood pressure is stubborn, I would encourage you to explore this path too.

By treating hypertension as the aggressive, silent threat it is, you can directly stabilize the foundation of your brain's health, protect its blood supply, and create a powerful environment for cognitive health.

CHAPTER 18

SOCIAL ISOLATION

Reversing Decline Through Social Connection

While diet, exercise, and stress management focus on your body's inner chemistry, social connection targets the heart of cognitive health by stimulating the brain and protecting your emotional well-being. Social isolation is a significant, yet often overlooked, risk factor for dementia. Reversing cognitive decline demands that you actively build and maintain a rich, engaged social life.

The Brain Science of Connection

Humans are fundamentally social creatures, and our brains are wired for interaction. When you are socially engaged, your brain is performing one of the most complex cognitive tasks possible.

1. Cognitive Demand and Reserve

Social interaction is a high-level cognitive workout that simultaneously engages multiple brain regions:

- Language and Communication: You are constantly processing spoken language, interpreting tone, generating responses, and recalling relevant information.

- Executive Function: You use planning, decision-making, and working memory to manage a conversation and navigate social situations.
- Theory of Mind: You must actively attempt to understand the thoughts, intentions, and beliefs of others, a sophisticated form of abstract reasoning.

This constant, demanding stimulation helps to build cognitive reserve, making your brain more resilient to the physical pathology of dementia.

2. The Stress and Inflammation Link

Social isolation acts as a form of chronic stress.

- Elevated Stress Hormones: Loneliness and isolation trigger the release of stress hormones like cortisol, which are toxic to the memory center (hippocampus).
- Chronic Inflammation: Isolation is linked to higher levels of systemic inflammation, which damages neurons, disrupts communication, and accelerates the accumulation of dementia-related proteins. Social connection is a powerful anti-inflammatory.

3. The Power of Purpose and Engagement

Feeling connected and having a sense of purpose through social roles (friend, grandparent, volunteer) is deeply protective. It reduces symptoms of depression and anxiety, which are themselves independent risk factors for dementia.

Your Prescription for Social Health

Social health is not about having hundreds of casual contacts; it's about nurturing a few meaningful, high-quality interactions. The goal is to move from passive existence to active engagement.

1. Structure Your Social Life (The "Social Routine")

Just as you schedule exercise, you must schedule interaction.

- The Daily Check-In: Make a commitment to genuinely connect with at least one person every day - a phone call, a video chat, or an in-person conversation.
- Join Structured Groups: Enroll in clubs, classes, or organizations where attendance is expected and interaction is mandatory. Good examples include a book club, a choir, a volunteer group, or a dance class.
- Focus on Shared Activity: Socializing over an activity (like playing a strategic game, learning a new language, or cooking a meal together) is more stimulating than simply watching TV side-by-side.

2. Cultivate Intergenerational Connections

Connecting with younger people provides unique cognitive and emotional benefits.

- Teach a Skill: Offer to teach a grandchild, neighbor, or community member a skill you possess—gardening, knitting, woodwork, or family history. The act of teaching demands high-level organization and memory recall.
- Volunteer with Youth: Programs that pair older adults with young students (tutoring, reading) are rewarding for both parties and provide a strong sense of purpose.

3. Embrace Technology for Connection

Do not let technology be a barrier; let it be a bridge.

- Master Video Calls: Learn to use platforms like Zoom, FaceTime, or Skype to maintain face-to-face contact with distant friends and family.
- Join Online Interest Groups: Participate in online forums, social media groups, or virtual book clubs dedicated to your hobbies. This provides mental stimulation and a sense of belonging without requiring you to leave home.

4. The Giving Paradox: Altruism and Health

Volunteering and altruistic activities are one of the best ways to combat social isolation.

- When you focus on helping others, you shift your mindset away from self-focus and stress.

- It provides an immediate sense of purpose and gratitude, both of which are strongly correlated with better physical and mental health outcomes.
- It places you in regular, meaningful contact with others who share a positive goal.

Reversing dementia is a journey that cannot be walked alone. By making social connection a deliberate, scheduled, and deeply valued part of your life, you are providing your brain with the powerful emotional and cognitive fuel it needs to heal and thrive.

CHAPTER 19

TOXINS

The cumulative burden of toxic exposure—from the air we breathe to the food we eat and the products we use—can silently erode brain function over decades. These toxins act as silent saboteurs, igniting chronic inflammation, inducing oxidative stress, and directly damaging the delicate machinery of your neurons. By identifying and reducing this toxic load, you introduce a powerful lever for reversing cognitive decline.

Major Toxic Culprits in Cognitive Decline

While the list of potential neurotoxins is vast, certain classes have been strongly implicated in the risk of dementia.

1. Heavy Metals

Heavy metals like lead, mercury, and cadmium are widespread and persistent. They are known neurotoxicants that can accumulate in the brain over time, even at low levels of exposure.

- Lead: A known neurotoxicant that can rapidly cross the blood-brain barrier. Chronic exposure has been associated with neuroinflammation, oxidative stress, and pathologies that mimic Alzheimer's disease, including amyloid-beta accumulation. Sources include old paint, contaminated water (especially from old pipes), and certain industrial exposures.

- Cadmium: Found in contaminated soil (which affects food crops), cigarette smoke, and some products. High levels are linked to decreased cognitive ability in older adults.
- Mercury: Considered highly dangerous to neurological health. Sources include certain types of seafood, dental amalgams, and contaminated water.

2. Mold and Mycotoxins

Exposure to water-damaged buildings can lead to the growth of mold that produces potent toxins called mycotoxins.

- Mycotoxins: These substances are highly lipophilic, allowing them to cross the blood-brain barrier and deposit in brain tissue. Case studies and small studies suggest that chronic mold and mycotoxin exposure can cause a constellation of neurological symptoms often referred to as "brain fog," including difficulty with memory, focus, and executive function.
- Mechanism of Harm: Mycotoxins drive pathogenic neuroinflammation, disrupt neurotransmitter metabolism, and induce significant oxidative stress in the brain.

3. Pesticides and Herbicides

Pesticides are chemicals explicitly designed to attack the nervous systems of insects, and mounting evidence shows they pose a serious threat to the human central nervous system as well.

- Organophosphates and Organochlorines: These classes of pesticides have been linked to an increased risk of neurodegenerative diseases, including Alzheimer's and Parkinson's disease. They often work by inhibiting crucial enzymes or inducing oxidative stress and inflammation in brain cells.
- Exposure Routes: The primary source of exposure is through the food chain (non-organic produce) and occupational exposure for agricultural workers. Long-term exposure to certain pesticides, even those banned decades ago like DDT, remains a concern as residues persist in the environment and human body fat.

4. Air Pollution

Exposure to polluted air is one of the most common and unavoidable environmental risks.

- Fine Particulate Matter: These tiny airborne particles (less than 2.5 micrometers in diameter) come from vehicle exhaust, industrial emissions, and wildfire smoke. They are so small that they can enter the bloodstream and directly damage the brain, leading to cerebrovascular damage and neuroinflammation.

- Increased Risk: High levels of air pollutants are associated with increased risk of cognitive decline, dementia, and a faster buildup of amyloid plaques in the brain.

5. Micro Plastics

Correlation with Dementia: A notable study from the University of New Mexico found that brain tissue from individuals with dementia had up to 10 times more plastic particles than those without the condition.

A Plan for Detoxification and Protection

Addressing the toxic burden is a critical pillar of any dementia reversal protocol. This involves a two-pronged strategy: reducing ongoing exposure and enhancing the body's natural ability to eliminate toxins.

Step 1: Reduce Toxin Exposure (The Prevention Plan)

- Purify Your Diet:
    - Filter Your Water: Invest in a high-quality water filter (carbon block or reverse osmosis) for drinking and cooking to remove heavy metals (like lead) and industrial contaminants.
    - Be Mindful of Seafood: Limit or avoid high-mercury fish and choose low-mercury options. https://www.nrdc.org/sites/default/files/walletcard.pdf

- Clean Your Air:
    - Use Air Purifiers: Place high-efficiency particulate air (HEPA) filters in your home, especially in the bedroom, to reduce fine particulate matter and mold spores.
    - Improve Ventilation: Ensure good ventilation, especially when cooking or using cleaning products.
    - Avoid Smoking/Secondhand Smoke: Cigarette smoke is a major source of toxins that directly harm the brain.
- Check Your Home Environment:
    - Test for Mold: If you suspect water damage or have chronic neurological symptoms, consider professional mold testing and remediation in your home.
    - Switch Cleaning Products: Replace conventional household and personal hygiene products with non-toxic, all-natural alternatives to reduce exposure to solvents and plastics.
    - Avoid food and drink in plastic, especially when heated.

Step 2: Support Detoxification and Elimination

Your body's primary detox organs—the liver, kidneys, and gut—need support to clear accumulated toxins.

- Liver Support: The liver is the main detox powerhouse. Give it the support it needs (all of these have already been mentioned)
    - Progesterone
    - Balanced nutrition
    - Minimize Polyunsaturated Fats
    - Check and address thyroid if needed
    - Lots of healthy sunshine
- Gut Health: The gut is the final exit for toxins cleared by the liver. Constipation or an unhealthy gut microbiome allows toxins to be reabsorbed.
    - Binders: In cases of known mycotoxin or certain heavy metal toxicity, a qualified practitioner may prescribe binding agents (such as charcoal, or certain fibers) to latch onto toxins in the gut and safely escort them out.
    - Insoluble Fiber: Ensure regular bowel movements and a healthy gut flora by including insoluble fiber in your diet. Well-cooked mushrooms, Bamboo shoots.

- Sweat Therapy: Infrared Saunas can be a powerful tool, as sweating is a proven route for the elimination of certain heavy metals and other chemicals stored in the body's fat tissues. Use with caution and consult a healthcare provider.
- Targeted Testing (If Applicable): If environmental toxin exposure is suspected, work with a practitioner to perform specialized testing, such as urine mycotoxin panels or heavy metal testing, to identify and quantify the specific toxic threats you need to address.

By taking proactive steps to clean up your environment and empower your body's natural detoxification systems, you can reduce chronic neuroinflammation, relieve the burden on your brain, and pave the way for cognitive repair and reversal.

CHAPTER 20

SMOKING AND ALCOHOL

I don't think I need to tell you that smoking is bad for your health and bad for your brain. So, I am going to skip telling you how it is bad for your brain. If you are still a smoker, I encourage you to keep trying the most effective things out there to help you quit. And keep quitting until it sticks.

Alcohol is a neurotoxin.

If you have any cognitive decline complete abstinence is strongly recommended to maximize the brain's ability to heal and repair.

CHAPTER 21

OBESITY

Obesity is a major accelerator of cognitive decline. Excess body fat is not just an aesthetic issue; it is a metabolic and endocrine organ that actively produces inflammatory compounds toxic to the brain.

The Deadly Trio: Obesity, Inflammation, and the Brain

Obesity contributes to cognitive decline through a dangerous synergy with other core risk factors, primarily insulin resistance and chronic inflammation.

1. Adipose Tissue as an Endocrine Organ

Excessive fat tissue (adipose tissue), particularly visceral fat stored around the organs, is biologically active. It functions like an aberrant endocrine gland that secretes pro-inflammatory signaling molecules called adipokines and cytokines.

- Chronic Neuro-Inflammation: These inflammatory messengers travel to the brain, easily cross the blood-brain barrier, and fuel chronic neuro-inflammation. This sustained inflammation damages neurons, disrupts synaptic function, and accelerates the buildup of toxic proteins like beta-amyloid and tau.
- Microglial Activation: The brain's resident immune cells, microglia, are constantly activated by this systemic

inflammation. When overactive, microglia shift from being protective to destructive, attacking and pruning healthy synapses, leading to cognitive loss.

2. The Insulin-Resistance Link

Obesity is a driver of insulin resistance, the condition some researchers call "Type 3 Diabetes".

- Metabolic Dysfunction: Fat cells interfere with the body's ability to respond to insulin, leading to chronically high insulin levels (hyperinsulinemia).
- Brain Energy Crisis: When the brain becomes insulin-resistant, it starves of its primary fuel (glucose), leading to impaired function in memory and executive centers. Weight loss directly improves insulin sensitivity, restoring energy supply to the brain.

3. Vascular Damage and Reduced Brain Volume

Obesity directly contributes to hypertension, high cholesterol, and sleep apnea, all of which compromise the brain's vascular health.

- Cerebral Hypoperfusion: The constellation of obesity-related vascular diseases reduces consistent blood flow to the brain (cerebral hypoperfusion). This lack of adequate oxygen and nutrients causes silent damage and accelerates the progression of vascular dementia.

- Brain Atrophy: Studies have shown a correlation between obesity and reduced volume in brain regions critical for memory and executive function, suggesting that obesity causes premature brain aging and atrophy.

Your Action Plan: Weight Loss as a Cognitive Strategy

For successful cognitive reversal, weight loss is not a side benefit - it is a treatment goal. The focus must be on reducing visceral fat and improving metabolic health, not just scale weight.

1. Strategic Dietary Intervention

The most effective approach is a clean balanced diet that provides all your nutrition.

I highly recommend Kate Deering's book, "How to Heal Your Metabolism".

https://amzn.to/4pIzJpj

2. Physical Activity for Metabolic Change

Exercise burns calories, but its primary cognitive benefit is its powerful effect on metabolic health and inflammation.

- Build Lean Muscle Mass: Resistance training (weightlifting, bodyweight exercises) is crucial. Muscle tissue is metabolically active and highly responsive to insulin, improving glucose clearance from the blood.

- Consistent Aerobic Activity: Daily brisk walking or other aerobic activity for at least 30 minutes improves blood flow to the brain and further enhances insulin sensitivity.

3. Sleep and Stress Management

These factors are deeply intertwined with weight gain and obesity.

- Cortisol and Belly Fat: Chronic stress leads to high cortisol, which promotes the storage of dangerous visceral fat around the abdomen. Effective stress management (meditation, deep breathing) is essential for controlling this fat storage pattern.
- Sleep and Appetite Hormones: Poor sleep disrupts the hormones that control hunger and satiety (ghrelin and leptin), leading to increased appetite and cravings. Prioritizing 7-9 hours of quality sleep nightly is a vital weight-control strategy.

By treating obesity as an endocrine disease that directly attacks the brain, you dismantle the chronic inflammatory and metabolic roadblocks to cognitive health, creating a fertile environment for your brain to heal and thrive.

CHAPTER 22

RED LIGHT

Red light therapy, also known as Photobiomodulation (PBM) or Low-Level Light Therapy (LLLT), is emerging as a promising, non-invasive, and drug-free approach to managing and potentially reversing aspects of cognitive decline and dementia. This therapy uses specific wavelengths of light, primarily red and near-infrared (NIR) light, to stimulate healing and cellular function within the brain. The preliminary evidence suggests it can offer significant benefits with minimal side effects, making it an exciting option in the fight against dementia.

The Powerhouse Effect: Mitochondria

The primary target for the light energy is the mitochondria, the "powerhouses" of your brain cells (neurons).

- Increased ATP Production: When light photons are absorbed by a specific enzyme in the mitochondria, it enhances the mitochondrial respiratory chain. This leads to a significant increase in the production of Adenosine Triphosphate (ATP), which is the main energy currency of the cell. In the brains of people with dementia, energy production is often impaired, and PBM aims to overcome this low ATP level.

- Reduced Oxidative Stress: The light helps to modulate Reactive Oxygen Species (ROS), which are linked to harmful oxidative stress—a key factor in neuronal damage and aging. By reducing this stress, PBM protects neurons and supports their longevity, potentially slowing the progression of neurodegenerative disorders.

Improving Brain Circulation

Red light improves circulation, enhancing the delivery of oxygen and essential nutrients to brain cells, as well as clearing waste products.

Neuroprotection and Repair

PBM has demonstrated significant neuroprotective effects, meaning it helps protect existing neurons from damage.

- New Cell Growth: There is emerging evidence that light therapy can promote neurogenesis (the creation of new neurons) and synaptogenesis (the formation of new connections between neurons), which is crucial for maintaining and restoring cognitive function.
- Anti-Inflammatory Action: Chronic inflammation in the brain is a major driver of dementia. PBM has shown the ability to exert an anti-inflammatory function, further protecting brain tissue from damage.

Clinical Benefits and Symptoms

Clinical studies, although still relatively small in number, have indicated that transcranial red and NIR light therapy can improve several key symptoms and cognitive measures in people with mild to moderate dementia:

Cognitive Function	Improvements in memory (long- and short-term), learning, and overall cognitive performance, as measured by standard tests like the Mini-Mental State Examination (MMSE) and the Alzheimer's Disease Assessment Scale-Cognitive (ADAS-Cog).
Sleep Patterns	Helps to reestablish a normal circadian rhythm (the body's internal clock), resulting in improved nighttime sleep and increased daytime wakefulness. This can reduce restlessness and agitation.
Behavioral Symptoms	Caregivers have reported that patients experience a reduction in agitation, aggression, anxiety, and wandering (often associated with 'sundowning'). It can also lead to an improved mood and energy level.
Activities of Daily Living	Patients have shown improvement in their ability to perform Activities of Daily Living (ADL).

Getting Started with Red Light Therapy

The Devices and Wavelengths

Red light therapy devices for the brain typically use Light Emitting Diodes (LEDs) or lasers to deliver light in two primary ranges:

1. Red Light (approx. 630 nm to 700 nm): Works well for more superficial tissue but also has systemic effects.

2. Near-Infrared (NIR) Light (approx. 800 nm to 1100 nm): This is generally considered optimal for brain treatment because the longer wavelengths penetrate the scalp and skull more efficiently to reach the deeper brain tissue.

Many devices designed for brain treatment are non-invasive headsets that deliver light transcranially (through the skull) and often include a nasal clip to deliver light intranasally.

Recommended Protocol

While protocols in clinical trials vary, a common therapeutic approach is generally:

- Frequency: Treatments are often administered daily or every other day (e.g., three times per week).
- Duration: Sessions are typically short, ranging from 6 to 20 minutes per session. The relative brevity and non-invasive nature of the therapy can make it easier for people with dementia to tolerate compared to long exposures to other forms of light therapy.
- Consistency: Like any other therapy for dementia, consistency is key. It can take a few weeks to notice changes in sleep and mood, and longer for cognitive improvements.

Safety and Consultation

Red light therapy is generally considered safe and remarkably free of side effects. However, it is essential to consult with a doctor or dementia specialist before beginning any new treatment to ensure it is appropriate for the individual and to discuss the specific device, intensity, and protocol.

CHAPTER 23

SLEEP

Good sleep is vital to brain health. The body is always ridding itself of toxins and waste products. For the brain, most of this happens when you sleep.

Here are some tips for quality sleep.

There is a long list of things that can disrupt your sleep and a long list of things that can help you sleep. Please keep experimenting until you find what works best for you and you find that Deep Restorative Sleep that you have been dreaming of.

1. Something salty sweet before bed. 6 ounces orange juice with a dash of salt. Adding 1 tablespoon collagen powder to it would be even better.

   6 ounces of warm milk with a teaspoon of honey and a pinch of salt.

   Fruit and Parmigiano Reggiano cheese.

   Have a salty sweet drink next to the bed if you wake up in the middle of the night.

2. Sleep in complete darkness. Use a sleep mask or completely black out all light.

3. A warm Epsom salt bath before bed.

4. Read or listen to relaxing music before bed.

5. Turn down the temperature in the bedroom.

6. Try a sound machine app.

7. Stop drinking caffeine 4-5 hours before bed.

8. Journal before bed.

9. Headspace app before bed.

10. Magnesium Glycinate before bed.

11. Binaural Beats: One of the best ways to improve the quality of your sleep is through listening to music that is specifically designed

to bring your brain from Beta (wide awake) to Alpha (awake but relaxed), Theta (REM sleep) and Delta (Deep sleep).

> Music to help you sleep:
> http://www.the-guided-meditation-site.com/free-meditation-music.html

12. Sunshine: Get at least ten minutes of sunshine first thing in the morning as close to sunrise as possible. If you are up before the sun, have the room well-lighted with incandescent or red light. Also get at least 15-45 minutes of mid-day sun without burning. The darker your skin is, the more sun you need.

13. Consistent Schedule: Do your best to go to sleep and wake up at the same time each day.

14. Electronics: Avoid electronics like TV, iPads and computer for at least a few hours before bed. If you must be in front of a screen, try blue-blocking optics like Gunnar glasses or set your screens so there is less blue light in the evening. http://www.gunnars.com/

15. Exercise: Participate in a fun exercise program. Exercise earlier in the day is probably best for those that are challenged getting to sleep.

16. Your Bed: Make sure that your mattress is comfortable.

17. Manage Stress: Create the habits that work best for you:

- Meditation
- Yoga

    - Thai Chi
    - Qigong
    - Walk
    - Hike
    - Swim
    - Flexibility and range of motion exercises
    - Breathing exercises
    - Music

18. If bathroom breaks have you up in the middle of the night, here is something you can try.

The part of the brain that is in charge of bladder and bowel control is also in charge of sensation of the lower legs.

I would test one of these each night just before bed. For 2 minutes on your lower legs try:

- Light touch
- Heavy touch
- Vibration
- Warm
- Cool
- Sharp (Safely) gently with the end of a paper clip

You could also test one leg at a time.

If any of these are dysfunctional or missing, I would encourage you to continue sensory retraining.

19. Eat less meat later in the day.

20. I do NOT recommend melatonin supplementation because it impairs mitochondrial energy production. It damages immunity by shrinking the thymus gland. It suppresses thyroid and progesterone and increases estrogen.

21. Keep the room well-lighted with incandescent or red light until you go to sleep.

22. Balance your blood sugar throughout the day. Eat frequently enough and have enough fat and protein with any carbs so that you keep your blood sugar in balance.

23. **Use carbon dioxide therapies.**
Carbon dioxide is an often-forgotten anti-stress substance. Many poor sleepers lack carbon dioxide, which is essential to energy metabolism and oxygenating the cells of the body (Bohr Effect). Carbon dioxide inhibits the release of serotonin (this is a good thing) and directly opposes stress-promoting lactic acid.

Those with hypothyroid tend to be deficient in CO2. Using carbon dioxide therapies during the day and at night such as bag breathing, drinking carbonated water, a baking soda bath, or consuming baking soda off the spoon or in a beverage can be useful. Buteyko breathing techniques like mouth taping or improving the control pause are other therapies to research.

24. Keep Polyunsaturated Fats (PUFA) down to 1 gram per 500 calories consumed.

25. **Be careful with fermented foods.**

Lactic acid is produced by cells during stress and also by bacteria in fermented foods. In either case, the liver is responsible for converting lactic acid into glucose. This process requires the use of fuel stored in the liver (glycogen). When available, glycogen is used during sleep to maintain the blood sugar so depleting it with fermented foods affects sleep quality and duration. To avoid this energy burden on the liver, reduction or elimination of fermented foods like kombucha, alcohol, yogurt, sauerkraut, and homemade fermented anything is a good idea. If you find yourself waking during the night, kick some of the fermented foods in your diet to curb for a while to see if your sleep improves.

26. Sleep Cocktail with one of the salty sweet drinks from above.

Niacinamide, 500mg (reduces anxiety)

https://amzn.to/4oi4aSy

Glycine, 1000mg (GABA receptor modulator)

https://amzn.to/4h9KCx9

Magnesium Glycinate, 400mg (suppresses neuroexcitation)

https://amzn.to/3W2Lji7

> That is 400 mg of "Magnesium Glycinate", NOT 400 mg of Magnesium.

If need be, you could double this dose and your sweet/salty drink for up to 3 weeks. Any more than that and you would want to re-evaluate how you are processing niacinamide.

CHAPTER 24

STRESS

Taming the Stress Monster

Chronic stress can accelerate the aging process in your brain. For those seeking to reverse cognitive decline, chronic stress management is a non-negotiable cornerstone of your recovery program. By learning to turn down the volume on your body's stress response, you can directly influence your brain's health, promoting healing and resilience.

The Hidden Cost of Chronic Stress on Your Brain

While a sudden, temporary stress response is essential for survival ("fight or flight"), chronic stress keeps your body in a state of constant, low-grade emergency. This prolonged state unleashes a cascade of biological changes that directly harm the brain, contributing to the pathology of dementia.

1. Cortisol: The Memory-Eroding Hormone

The primary driver of the chronic stress-dementia link is the stress hormone cortisol, released by the hypothalamic-pituitary-adrenal (HPA) axis.

- Hippocampal Damage: Sustained high levels of cortisol are neurotoxic, particularly to the hippocampus—the brain's main memory center. Cortisol exposure can cause neurons in the hippocampus to shrink and new neuron formation (neurogenesis) to decrease, essentially eroding the very structure responsible for forming new memories.

- Glucose Blockade: Excess cortisol also interferes with the brain's ability to utilize glucose for energy, starving brain cells and impairing their function.

2. Chronic Inflammation

Stress is a significant trigger for inflammation throughout the body and brain.

- Immune System Dysregulation: Chronic stress dysregulates the immune system, leading to the sustained release of pro-inflammatory chemicals, or cytokines, in the brain.
- Neuro-Inflammation: This chronic neuro-inflammation damages neurons, disrupts communication between brain cells, and accelerates the accumulation of damaging proteins, such as beta-amyloid plaques and tau tangles, which are hallmarks of Alzheimer's disease.

3. Cellular Stress and Neuron Death

New research suggests that protein aggregates (the clumps that form plaques and tangles) may not directly kill brain cells, but rather prevent the cell's natural stress response from turning off. This perpetual, unchecked cellular stress response is what ultimately leads to neuron death. By managing chronic stress, you support your cells' ability to maintain a healthy balance and "silence" this toxic stress signal.

Stress Management: Your Cognitive Tool Kit

The good news is that the systems compromised by chronic stress—cortisol levels, inflammation, and cellular resilience—are highly modifiable. By integrating consistent stress-reducing practices, you create a powerful, neuroprotective environment for your brain to heal and rebuild.

1. Mind-Body Practices

These techniques are specifically designed to calm the nervous system and lower cortisol.

Technique	Cognitive Benefit	How to Start
Mindfulness & Meditation	Reduces cortisol, improves focus and attention, and promotes structural changes in the prefrontal cortex related to emotional regulation.	Start with just 5-10 minutes daily. Use guided apps or simply focus on your breath.
Deep Abdominal Breathing	Activates the parasympathetic nervous system ("rest and digest"), directly counteracting the stress response.	Practice 4-7-8 breathing: Inhale for 4 seconds, hold for 7 seconds, exhale for 8 seconds. Repeat 5-10 times.
Yoga and Tai Chi	Combines gentle movement, deep breathing, and meditation to lower stress hormones and improve mind-body connection.	Look for a beginner Hatha or Restorative yoga class, or an online Tai Chi tutorial.

2. The Power of Movement

Physical activity is one of the most potent natural stress relievers.

- Release Endorphins: Exercise releases endorphins, natural mood boosters and pain relievers that override stress signals.
- Burn Off Cortisol: It helps metabolize and clear excess stress hormones from your bloodstream.
- Improve Sleep: Regular exercise is a key factor in improving sleep quality, which is critical for the brain's waste-clearing glymphatic system to remove neurotoxic proteins like amyloid. Aim for 150 minutes of moderate cardio and 2-3 strength training sessions per week.

3. Prioritizing Rest and Recovery

Lack of quality sleep is both a symptom and a cause of chronic stress, and a significant risk factor for cognitive decline.

- Establish a Consistent Sleep Schedule: Go to bed and wake up around the same time, even on weekends, to regulate your body's natural sleep-wake cycle.
- Optimize Your Sleep Environment: Ensure your bedroom is dark, cool, and quiet. Avoid screens (phones, tablets, TV) for at least one hour before bed, as the blue light suppresses the sleep hormone melatonin.

- Use the Bed Only for Sleep and Intimacy: This helps condition your brain to associate the bed with rest, not stress or work.

4. Cultivate Connection and Joy

Social isolation and loneliness are powerful stressors that negatively impact brain health.

- Increase Social Engagement: Regularly interact with friends, family, and community. Social contact provides distraction, emotional support, and reduces the feeling of being overwhelmed. Consider volunteering—helping others is a proven way to boost resilience and reduce stress.
- Schedule "Me Time": Intentionally set aside time for hobbies and activities that bring you joy and a sense of calm. This could be listening to music, gardening, reading, or creative arts. Laughter, in particular, has been shown to reduce cortisol.

5. Cognitive Reframing and Professional Support

How you think about stress is as important as the events themselves.

- Identify Your Stressors: Keep a journal to track what triggers your stress, how it makes you feel, and your typical reaction. Recognizing patterns is the first step to changing them.

- Practice Cognitive Reframing: Use techniques from Cognitive Behavioral Therapy (CBT) to challenge and reframe negative or catastrophic thoughts. Focus on setting realistic expectations and accepting situations you cannot change.
- Seek Professional Help: If your stress feels overwhelming, or is manifesting as chronic anxiety or depression, consult a mental health professional. Therapy can provide effective, personalized strategies for managing deep-seated stress responses.

The Takeaway

You have the power to turn down the dial on the stress response that is silently damaging your brain. By actively integrating stress management—through conscious relaxation, regular exercise, quality sleep, and social connection - you are not just improving your mood; you are directly modifying a key risk factor for dementia. Embracing these practices creates an optimal environment in your brain for healing, promoting neurogenesis, and moving you further along the path to cognitive health.

CHAPTER 25

SUPPORT

The Power of Community: Building Your Support System

The journey to reverse dementia is not a solitary one. It demands rigorous lifestyle changes, emotional resilience, and relentless optimism, which can be exhausting for both the individual seeking reversal and their caregivers. Building a robust support system is, therefore, not a luxury - it is an essential component of the therapeutic protocol. This chapter will guide you in harnessing the strength of community to sustain your efforts and maximize your chances of success.

Why Support is a Non-Negotiable Intervention

A strong support system acts as a protective shield against the key enemies of cognitive health: stress, isolation, and burnout.

1. Combating the Stress of Change

Implementing a healthy brain/dementia reversing lifestyle can feel overwhelming.

- Shared Accountability: A partner, family member, or health coach can provide the accountability needed to stay consistent with the program, especially on difficult days.

- Lowering Cortisol: Having a trusted circle of people to talk to reduces feelings of anxiety and stress. Managing stress directly lowers the neurotoxic hormone cortisol, protecting your memory center.

2. Defeating Isolation and Depression

Dementia is often accompanied by social withdrawal, and social isolation itself is a major risk factor.

- Active Engagement: A support system ensures regular, mandatory social contact, which combats isolation and provides the high-level cognitive stimulation necessary to build neuroplasticity.
- Mood Regulation: Support networks provide the emotional buffer needed to prevent or treat depression, which can otherwise sabotage motivation and accelerate cognitive decline.

3. Preventing Caregiver Burnout

This journey places significant demands on caregivers and partners. If the caregiver burns out, the entire system collapses, and the protocol can fail. Support is a two-way street that must include relief and resources for the entire team.

Building Your Multi-Tiered Support Network

Your support system should be structured like an inverted pyramid, with personalized, intimate support at the top, broadened by specialized professionals and community resources.

1. Tier 1: The Inner Circle (The "Why")

These are the people whose lives are most intertwined with yours. They provide emotional core and daily logistical help.

- The Partner: This is the most crucial member—a spouse, child, or close friend who is fully committed to learning the protocol and helping with daily tasks (meal preparation, exercise reminders, appointment scheduling). Their commitment must be unwavering.
- The Family Team: Educate all close family members on the program's rationale. Even if they don't follow the full protocol, their understanding and non-sabotaging behavior (e.g., not offering tempting foods) are essential.
- Peer Support: Connect with others who are actively engaged in reversing cognitive decline. Sharing successes and struggles with peers who understand the unique challenges provides validation and motivation.

2. Tier 2: The Professional Team (The "How")

These experts provide the specialized knowledge required to personalize and manage the complexities of reversing dementia.

- Get the professional help that you need and make sure they are on board and supportive of you reversing dementia.

3. Tier 3: Community Resources (The "Buffer")

These groups provide structured activities, emotional respite, and a wider sense of belonging.

- Support Groups: Local or virtual groups for dementia caregivers or those with Mild Cognitive Impairment (MCI). These offer invaluable emotional understanding and practical advice.
- Structured Activities: Groups like book clubs, community choirs, volunteer organizations, or adult day programs (for socialization and stimulation) provide structure and reduce the burden on the primary caregiver.
- Respite Care: Utilizing temporary, scheduled care services allows the primary caregiver to take necessary breaks. Respite is not a failure; it is a critical act of self-preservation that prevents burnout and ensures the continuity of the entire reversal effort.

Your Support System Checklist

To effectively harness the power of support, perform these three actions immediately:

1. Delegate: Look at your protocol list and assign a minimum of three tasks to your inner circle (e.g., "Partner manages all

dinner meal prep," "Daughter handles supplement reordering," "Friend calls for 10-minute check-in daily").

2. Schedule: Block out specific time each week for social connection and caregiver respite. Treat these appointments with the same importance as a doctor's visit.
3. Communicate: Hold an honest family meeting to discuss the diagnosis, the reversal plan, and the specific needs of the person with cognitive decline and the primary caregiver. Clear, consistent communication prevents misunderstandings and garners true cooperation.

By consciously surrounding yourself with a committed team, you ensure the emotional and logistical stability required to sustain your reversing dementia program, turning a difficult challenge into a collective mission.

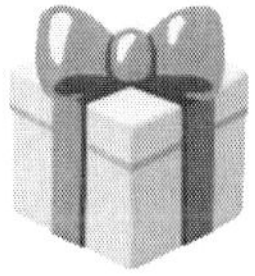

CHAPTER 26

DENTAL HEALTH

There is a growing body of research suggesting a strong link between dental health and dementia. While the exact relationship is still being studied, here's a breakdown of the key connections:

1. The Role of Inflammation and Bacteria

Gum Disease (Periodontitis): This is the most significant link. Periodontal disease is a chronic inflammatory condition caused by bacteria in the mouth. These bacteria and the inflammatory molecules they produce can enter the bloodstream, travel to the brain, and contribute to neuroinflammation.

Specific Bacteria: Researchers have identified certain oral bacteria, particularly Porphyromonas gingivalis, as a potential culprit. This bacterium, a major cause of gum disease, has been found in the brains of people with Alzheimer's disease.

Beta-Amyloid Plaques: Some studies suggest that the brain may produce beta-amyloid plaques—a hallmark of Alzheimer's—as a defense mechanism in response to these bacterial infections.

2. The Impact of Tooth Loss

Higher Risk: Studies have found that older adults with more missing teeth have a significantly higher risk of cognitive impairment and dementia. The risk appears to increase with each lost tooth.

Nutritional Deficiencies: Tooth loss can lead to difficulties with chewing, which might result in a poor diet and nutritional deficiencies that affect brain function.

Social and Psychological Factors: Tooth loss can also be an indicator of lower socioeconomic status or a lack of access to healthcare, which are also independently linked to a higher risk of dementia. Interestingly, one study found that people who had missing teeth but used dentures did not have a significantly higher risk of dementia, which suggests that the ability to chew and maintain proper nutrition may be a key factor.

What This Means for Prevention and Care

While more research is needed to establish a definitive causal link, the evidence highlights the importance of good dental hygiene for overall health and well-being, especially as we age. Maintaining a consistent routine of brushing, flossing, mouthwash, oil pulling, and regular dental check-ups may be a simple yet important way to help protect cognitive function.

CHAPTER 27

LITHIUM

Recent studies, particularly a landmark study from Harvard Medical School published in *Nature* in late August 2025, are providing strong evidence that lithium may play a crucial role in preventing and even reversing memory loss, particularly in the context of Alzheimer's disease.

Here's a breakdown of the key findings and the broader scientific context:

The Harvard Study (August 2025)

- Natural Brain Function: The study, led by Dr. Bruce Yankner, found for the first time that lithium exists naturally in the human brain in small amounts. It appears to be essential for normal brain function and cognitive resilience.
- Lithium Deficiency and Alzheimer's: The researchers discovered that people with mild cognitive impairment and advanced Alzheimer's disease have significantly lower levels of lithium in their brains compared to cognitively healthy individuals. They also found that toxic amyloid plaques in the brain bind to lithium, effectively "depleting" it and preventing it from performing its essential functions.

- Reversing Memory Loss in Mice: In trials on mouse models of Alzheimer's, researchers found they could reverse the disease, prevent brain cell damage, and restore memory loss by administering a low dose of a lithium compound called lithium orotate. This form of lithium was particularly effective because it was not bound by the amyloid plaques.
- Low-Dose vs. High-Dose: The study highlighted the efficacy of a very low dose of lithium orotate—one-thousandth the clinical dose of lithium carbonate used for bipolar disorder—which was effective without causing toxicity. This addresses a major concern with traditional lithium treatment, which has a narrow therapeutic window and can cause significant side effects at higher doses.

Broader Scientific Evidence and Mechanisms

The Harvard study builds upon a growing body of research that supports lithium's neuroprotective properties.

- Neuroprotective Effects: Numerous studies have shown that lithium has a range of neuroprotective effects. It can help reduce the formation of amyloid plaques and tau tangles, which are hallmarks of Alzheimer's. It also helps to enhance neurogenesis (the creation of new neurons) and synaptic plasticity (the brain's ability to form new connections).
- Inhibiting GSK-3β: A key mechanism by which lithium is thought to work is by inhibiting an enzyme called glycogen

synthase kinase-3β (GSK-3β). This enzyme is implicated in the development of Alzheimer's disease, and its inhibition by lithium appears to be crucial for its therapeutic effects on the brain.

- Population Studies: Several epidemiological studies have found a correlation between higher levels of trace lithium in public drinking water and lower rates of dementia in the population. While these studies show correlation, not causation, they support the idea that even microdoses of lithium may have a protective effect over a lifetime.
- Clinical Trials: While the most recent and promising research has been in animal models, there have been some human clinical trials. A meta-analysis of small, placebo-controlled trials found that lithium significantly slowed cognitive decline in patients with mild cognitive impairment or Alzheimer's. However, these results are considered preliminary, and more extensive, long-term human trials are needed.

Important Considerations

- Lithium Carbonate vs. Lithium Orotate: It's important to differentiate between the forms of lithium. Lithium carbonate is the high-dose psychiatric medication with a risk of significant side effects. Lithium orotate is a dietary supplement that has shown promise in recent studies at much lower doses. The Harvard study specifically found that lithium orotate was more effective at evading amyloid plaques than lithium carbonate.

- More Research is Needed: Despite the exciting findings, it's crucial to understand that the research is still in its early stages. The results in animal models do not always translate to humans. Large-scale, well-controlled clinical trials in humans are the next critical step to definitively determine the efficacy and safety of low-dose lithium supplementation for memory loss and Alzheimer's prevention.
- Consult a Healthcare Professional: Lithium, in any form, can have effects on the body. Anyone considering lithium supplementation should consult with a healthcare professional to discuss the potential risks and benefits.

The Harvard Study (August 2025) highlighted the efficacy of a very low dose of lithium orotate for cognitive health - one-thousandth the clinical dose of lithium carbonate used for bipolar disorder.

Based on typical clinical doses of lithium carbonate for bipolar disorder, the dose of lithium orotate for cognitive health would be between 1.2 mg and 1.8 mg per day.

The key takeaway from the Harvard study is that these very small, "microdoses" of lithium orotate were effective without the toxic side effects associated with the much higher doses of lithium carbonate.

Caveats: Important Considerations

- Individual Variation: Everyone's body processes supplements differently. The Harvard study noted that a microdose was effective for mice, but this may not be the case for all humans. Individual health conditions, genetics, and diet can all affect how lithium orotate is absorbed and utilized.
- Interaction with Medications: Lithium can interact with a wide range of medications, even at low doses. It is especially critical to check with your healthcare provider before supplementing with lithium orotate if you are taking:
    - Diuretics (water pills): These can affect the kidneys' ability to clear lithium, leading to a build-up of the mineral.
    - NSAIDs: Nonsteroidal anti-inflammatory drugs like ibuprofen can increase lithium levels.
    - ACE Inhibitors: Medications for high blood pressure can also increase lithium levels.
- Underlying Health Conditions: Lithium, in any form, is processed by the kidneys. Individuals with pre-existing kidney or thyroid conditions should not take lithium orotate without strict medical supervision. It is also

contraindicated for those with certain heart conditions (e.g., Brugada syndrome).

CHAPTER 28

LAUGHTER

The Best Medicine: Harnessing Laughter

Laughter isn't just a pleasant side effect of joy; it's a potent, physiological intervention with direct anti-inflammatory, stress-busting, and cognitive-boosting effects.

The Biochemistry of a Good Laugh

When you laugh - whether genuine or self-induced - your body experiences a cascade of beneficial biochemical and neurological changes that directly counteract the mechanisms of cognitive decline.

1. The Stress Hormone Antidote

Laughter is a direct and immediate countermeasure to the stress response.

- Lowering Cortisol: A hearty laugh reduces the levels of cortisol (the neurotoxic stress hormone) and adrenaline. By calming the hypothalamic-pituitary-adrenal (HPA) axis, laughter protects the hippocampus (the memory center) from stress-induced atrophy.
- Boosting Endorphins: Laughter triggers the release of endorphins, the body's natural feel-good chemicals. These

not only elevate mood and reduce pain but also help create a positive emotional state that is conducive to learning and neuroplasticity.

2. The Anti-Inflammatory Effect

Chronic inflammation is a key driver of dementia. Laughter helps turn down the body's inflammatory dial.

- Immune Modulation: Laughter improves the function of the immune system by increasing the production of T-cells and natural killer cells. This stronger immune response is better able to manage chronic, low-grade inflammation throughout the body and brain.
- Vascular Health: Laughter improves the function of the endothelium (the lining of blood vessels), promoting vasodilation (widening of the vessels) and improving blood flow. This direct benefit to cerebral blood flow is crucial for delivering oxygen and nutrients to the brain and protecting against vascular dementia.

3. Cognitive and Social Stimulation

Laughter and humor are highly complex cognitive activities that engage multiple brain regions.

- Whole-Brain Workout: Understanding a joke requires rapid processing, abstract thought, and recall of context—a true whole-brain exercise. This kind of spontaneous, complex activity supports cognitive reserve.

- Strengthening Social Bonds: Laughter is deeply tied to social connection. Shared humor strengthens relationships, reduces feelings of isolation, and provides a powerful source of emotional resilience.

Your Prescription for Joyful Reversal

Making laughter a therapeutic tool requires conscious effort and integration into your daily routine.

1. Curate a Daily Humor Dose

Do not leave joy to chance. Intentionally seek out humor every day.

- Visual and Auditory Aids: Watch 10-15 minutes of stand-up comedy, a funny movie clip, or a pet video. Schedule this time just as you would schedule exercise.
- Reading Material: Keep a collection of joke books, humorous essays, or silly cartoons easily accessible.

2. Connect with Your Funny Bone (and Others')

Integrate humor into your social interactions for maximum benefit.

- The Funny Friend: Prioritize spending time with people who have a good sense of humor and who make you laugh. Their energy is contagious and therapeutically beneficial.
- Share Humor: Actively share jokes, funny stories, or observations. The act of recounting a funny moment and

seeing someone else laugh is a powerful mood and cognitive booster.

- Play and Lightheartedness: Engage in playful, lighthearted activities. This might mean playing a silly game, deliberately telling a bad joke, or simply making funny observations about daily life.

3. Adopt a Humorous Perspective (Cognitive Reframing)

Humor is often a matter of perspective and a fantastic tool for stress management.

- Self-Deprecating Humor: Learn to laugh at your own minor errors or frustrations. This reframes an imperfection not as a source of stress or failure, but as a moment of levity.
- Look for Absurdity: Train your mind to spot the ridiculous or absurd elements in stressful or frustrating situations. This cognitive shift can turn anxiety into amusement.

Laughter is a universal language of well-being. By embracing it as a formal component of your dementia reversal protocol, you unlock a powerful, natural, and enjoyable pathway to reduce inflammation, tame stress, and strengthen the neural networks of your brain.

CHAPTER 29

HABITS AND ROUTINES

Harnessing Habits and Routines

Reversing dementia is not achieved through sudden, heroic efforts, but through the relentless consistency of small, positive choices. Habits and routines are the invisible architecture that support this consistency. For individuals experiencing cognitive decline, establishing predictable, supportive routines is particularly crucial, as they reduce cognitive load, conserve mental energy, and ensure the daily execution of your entire therapeutic protocol.

The Brain Science of Routine

The brain loves predictability. Routine allows essential tasks to shift from the energy-intensive prefrontal cortex (the thinking, planning part) to the basal ganglia (the automatic behavior center).

1. Reducing Cognitive Load

Cognitive decline makes planning, decision-making, and remembering complex sequences incredibly difficult.

- Automaticity: When an action becomes a routine (e.g., taking supplements at the same time every morning, walking after every dinner), it requires virtually no conscious effort or memory recall. The mental energy saved can then be redirected toward challenging cognitive exercises or learning.

- Conserving Executive Function: Executive function (planning, organizing, initiating tasks) is often the first cognitive domain to weaken. Routines minimize the need to constantly plan, preserving this limited resource for times when it is genuinely needed.

2. Entraining Biological Rhythms

Many dementia reversal protocols, such as optimizing sleep and managing stress, depend on regulating the body's internal clocks (circadian rhythms).

- Hormonal Regulation: Consistent routines for waking up, eating, and sleeping help synchronize the release of crucial hormones stabilizing mood, energy, and sleep quality—all essential for brain repair.

Structure and Simplicity

A successful routine for cognitive health is highly structured, yet flexible enough to adapt to occasional disruptions.

1. The Anchor Habit

Every effective routine needs a non-negotiable anchor—a simple, powerful habit that ensures the entire system doesn't unravel.

- Sleep/Wake Time: The most powerful anchor. Set a strict, non-negotiable bedtime and wake-up time, even on weekends. This is the foundation for all hormonal and metabolic healing.

- The Morning Stack: Immediately upon waking, link a few key behaviors together: Healthy morning drink, Take morning supplements, Go outside for light exposure. Once the first domino (waking) falls, the others follow automatically.

2. The Integrated Protocol Schedule

Integrate the necessary therapeutic actions into existing parts of your day to ensure adherence.

Protocol Component	Routine Integration	Benefit
Physical Exercise	Always walk for 30 minutes immediately after dinner (or another specific meal).	Enhances insulin sensitivity; improves cerebral blood flow.
Cognitive Exercise	Always read/do puzzles for 20 minutes immediately before dinner.	Ensures consistency; separates cognitive work from screen time.
Supplementation	Use a pillbox and link supplement intake to specific meals	Prevents missed doses; ensures proper absorption.
Stress Management	Always meditate for 10 minutes after breakfast.	Makes stress relief a daily, automatic priority.

3. Simplify the Environment

For individuals with cognitive decline, the environment must be simplified to reduce friction and minimize errors.

- Clutter Control: A cluttered environment causes visual overstimulation and increases cognitive load. Keep workspaces and living areas clean and organized.
- Visual Cues: Use visual cues instead of relying on memory. Place running shoes by the door for your walk, put supplements next to the breakfast plate, or use color-coded systems for clothes or tasks.
- Automate Decisions: Make as many decisions as possible ahead of time. Prep healthy meals on Sunday, lay out clothes the night before, and create a single, designated spot for keys and wallet.

By purposefully constructing a supportive framework of habits and routines, you turn the challenging demands of the dementia reversal protocol into a consistent, automatic flow, creating the sustained momentum required for genuine cognitive healing.

CHAPTER 30

REVIEW

I hope you agree that this book should not just be a onetime read, but would rather be best reviewed again, and again, ... continuing to build and improve your healthy brain lifestyle.

There is a wealth of knowledge in this book, but it is not everything on brain health and this is a rapidly developing topic. I encourage you to be a lifelong student of this subject, whether that is through working with me or learning from others that know cognitive decline, dementia, and Alzheimer's can be prevented and when starting soon enough, can be reversed.

CHAPTER 31

PERSONALIZE

There are now at least a few multi-faceted lifestyles approaches to preventing and reversing cognitive decline/dementia/Alzheimer's that are rather effective.

And I have no doubt that they would be even more effective if they were personalized.

There is no one size fits all diet, workout, or anything.

There isn't even a specific diet or workout that will work for you through the different phases of your life.

Keep reflecting, evaluating, and testing to find what works for you.

Personalize your brain workouts. Computer-based brain exercises can be great, but make sure to take this into the real world too. In what areas does your brain need more work or more stimulation? Social? Memory? Attention? Processing Speed? Relaxation? Quality Movement? …? Your brain may also need less stimulation in some areas.

If you need any help with any of this, let me know.

I commend you for getting this far and encourage you to be patient and persistent in your continued journey. When you inevitably get off track, be kind to yourself and back on track ASAP.

REVIEW REQUEST

Help Spread the Word

If you haven't already, please take this moment to leave a review on Amazon.

https://bit.ly/ReverseDementia

Thank You

BONUSES

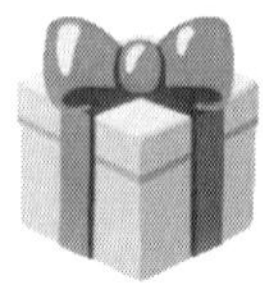

Your 7-Day QuickStart Guide to Reversal of Cognitive Decline…

& much more

Get Instant Access Now

https://youcanreversedementia.com/quickstart

ACKNOWLEDGEMENTS

This would not have been possible without you.

Dr. Eric Cobb of Z-Health Performance Solutions

https://zhealtheducation.com/

Zacharian Salazar of MTG (Meander Toward Greatness)

ZachariahSalazar@gmail.com

Bryan Thomas of BRAINHAB

https://www.brainhab.com/

About the Author

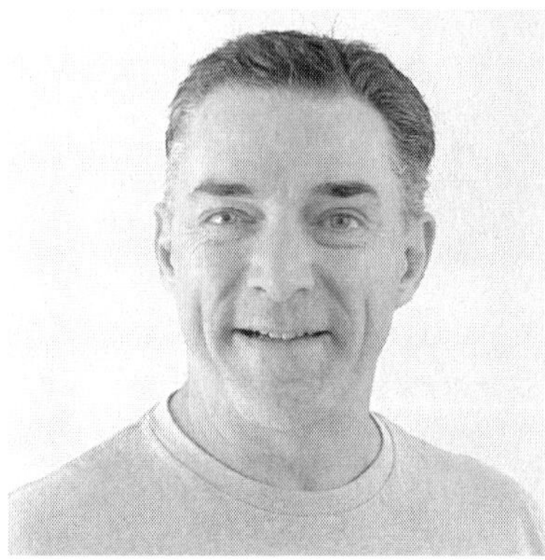

Paul Wayne Bowman is on a mission to make sure everyone knows that You Can Reverse Dementia. He is dedicated to empowering individuals and caregivers with the proven, science- backed strategies for maximizing cognitive function. Driven by a personal high-risk profile, including a strong family history and over 100 concussions, Paul is a bestselling author and neuro coach helping people improve cognition, function, balance, movement, mobility, and joint pain through applied neurology.

Visit his website at:

https://youcanreversedementia.com/about-paul/

All inquiries for podcast appearances, video shows, and speaking can be sent to paul@youcanreversedementia.com

OTHER BOOKS BY PAUL WAYNE BOWMAN

Available at https://youcanreversedementia.com/books/

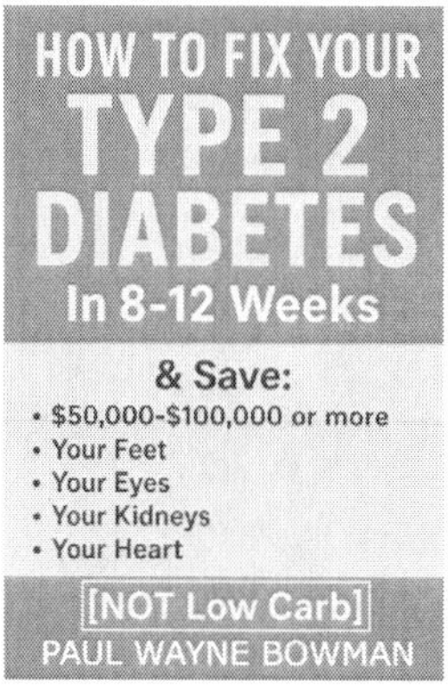

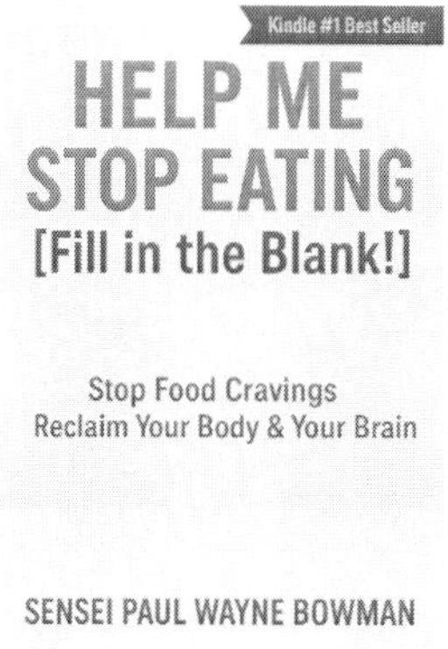

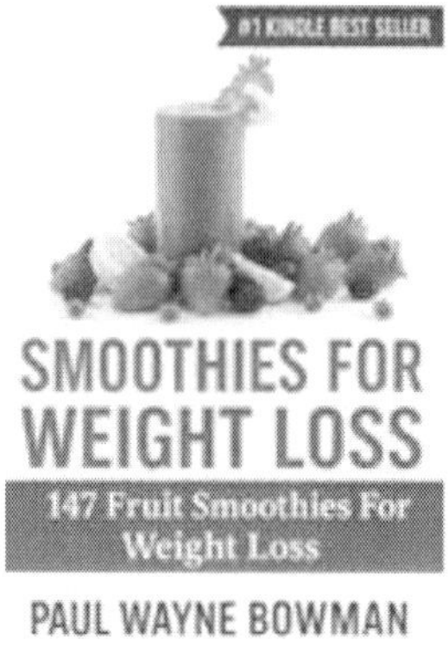

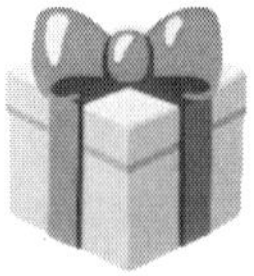

Your 7-Day QuickStart Guide to Reversal of Cognitive Decline

Get Instant Access Now

https://youcanreversedementia.com/quickstart

Made in United States
North Haven, CT
10 November 2026

22088256R00076